I0423865

PALEO DIET

The Top 110 Delicious Paleo Diet Recipes to Lose Weight, Boost Energy, Live Healthy, and Satisfy Your Hunger!

by

Hannah Parkes

Copyright & Disclaimer:

Adherence to all applicable laws and regulations, including international, federal, state, and local governing professional licensing, business practices, advertising, and all other aspects of doing business in the US, Canada, or any other jurisdiction is the sole responsibility of the reader or purchaser.

Neither the author nor the publisher assumes any responsibility or liability whatsoever on the behalf of the purchaser or reader of these materials.

Any perceived slight of any individual or organizations is purely unintentional.

Introduction

The Paleo diet: it's all the rage. Seems like everyone is doing it, and they're all crazy healthy. They probably do CrossFit, or run marathons, or bust out a thousand crunches a day. You've heard that if you're on the Paleo diet, you have to eat raw eggs and worship kale. If you touch sweets, you spontaneously combust.

Luckily, most of that is totally false. A Paleo diet can work for *anyone*: busy parents, people who have always had trouble eating well, workers stuck in an office eighty hours a week, whomever! Paleo is not just for athletes (though it will boost your energy and make workouts easier). This e-book will explain the science behind a Paleo diet, why it will help you be healthier, and how you can easily and safely take on a Paleo lifestyle without driving yourself insane.

You'll find strategies for getting started, including how to avoid common mistakes, tips for navigating the grocery store, how to make Paleo affordable, and foolproof-beginner recipes.

With the easy-to-understand guidance in this book and the included 30-day beginner's plan, you'll be off living your best life in no time.

Table of Contents

Chapter 1 What is a Paleo diet, and how does it work?

You're heard the hype, but what in the blazes IS the Paleo diet?

In the beginning...

First off, "Paleo" is short for "Paleolithic:" *Paleo* basically means "old" and *lithic* is based on the Greek word for stone. There you go: the Paleolithic era was the Stone Age, 2.5 million years ago, when our earliest human ancestors started to get fancy and invent tools.

Why do we care about the Stone Age, and what does it have to do with a diet? Because nutritionists have determined that our earliest human ancestors and *what they ate* should be foundation for the Paleo diet

You see, even though 2.5 million years sounds like a really, really long time ago, for the human body, it's just the blink of an eye.

Not all that much has changed for us in those years, and while the varieties of available foods has exploded, the idea is our bodies are somewhat stuck in the past. We still process food in similar ways, and if that's the case, why are we getting crazy and dumping all these exotic preservatives, sugars, and chemicals into our system? And when we do that, why are we surprised when we don't feel so great afterward?

Playing to our evolutionary strengths

The idea behind the Paleo diet is that we need to get back to our diet roots. A couple million years ago, we were eating fruit and vegetables and meat; it was simple, but we could get everything we needed and then some from those basic ingredients. There were no processed foods, fewer cereal grains, no added sugar, and no preservatives.

Nowadays, we've cleverly invented things like potato chips and frozen dinners and pizza, which taste *great* and are easy to get, but aren't great for us. They pile on the pounds and make us predisposed to heart diseases and diabetes, among other nasty illnesses.

A Paleo diet recommends you give up those modern extras, like corn syrup and nitrates. (Diet or no, does it really sound all that bad to axe those things?)

Let's simplify, simplify, simplify, and get you feeling great by going back to basics. Don't be nervous about having supposedly fewer ingredients to play with—there are many ways to make your meals delicious without adding a ton of unhealthy condiments and fillers, and we'll show you show later in the guide.

Science

(For the sake of accuracy, a quick note: technically speaking, our ancient ancestors, despite being hunter-gatherers, most likely did have access to cereal grains and other more "modern" foods; however, for the purpose of this guide, we're going to stick with the more recent nutritionist-developed definition of a Paleo diet that was presented above. If you'd like to learn more about the hunter-gatherer eating profile, check out this Scientific American article.)

Will a Paleo diet work for me?

Now you know the history of the Paleo diet, and you might be a little intimidated. That's OK—it's a lot to take in, but don't abandon ship yet. No matter where you're starting, you can make a Paleo diet work for you.

One of the biggest things to remember is that you can start slowly with this. In fact, especially if a more basic diet is something you're not used to, *gradually* eliminate those non-Paleo foods. The more radical the change, the harder it is to sustain, and the more likely you are to burn out and go back to your old habits.

That being said, if you're feeling really good and want to immediately rid your pantry and fridge of all non-Paleo items, go for it!

Some people have a much easier time going cold turkey than doing a step-by-step program.

While a Paleo diet has the wonderful effect of slimming you down, decreasing bloat and giving you more energy, it's most effective when it's not used only for weight loss. Eating Paleo is more than a diet—it's a lifestyle change that will reward you with a leaner physique, more energy, and greater mental clarity.

How and why does the Paleo diet work?

The bottom line of a Paleo diet is, choose foods whose purpose is to nourish your body. If a food has empty calories and no nutrients, it has no purpose, and you do not need to eat it.

(Note: if you're familiar with nutrition and don't need a refresher on how our bodies process energy, skip to the next section.)

We've learned a little bit about why Paleo is effective but let's dig a little bit deeper into the mechanisms behind its success, and why a Paleo diet focuses on specific kinds of foods.

Reviewing some basic biology and foundations of nutrition shows how your body processes nutrients, which will help you make sense of what you're eating and why:

The Human Torch:

All of your pieces and parts, from your brain to your toes, are powered by the energy you derive from food. Food comes in three broad categories: fats, proteins, and carbohydrates. All of those things are broken down, some more quickly than others, into a kind of really basic sugar (if you're interested, that basic sugar is called ATP) that's used to power all your cells.

Think of fats as a slow-burning candle, protein as a lighter, and carbohydrates as a match.

Fats: Did you know your brain is basically a big ball of fat? Your cells need fats in order to create their membranes. Too little fat is downright unhealthy. Embrace fat. (The right kinds of fat, of course. More on that later.) Fat is a slow burner (remember the candle) so once you have a lot of fat to burn, getting rid of it takes time. Fat is not the enemy—empty carbohydrates are.

Proteins: Proteins are the jack-of-all-trade in your body. Eating protein is really important because they contain amino acids, AKA the basis of everything important in your body, including your DNA, and we can't produce those amino acids by ourselves. Like a lighter, proteins provide longer-term services and you can pull them out of your pocket when you need them. Proteins build muscle fibers, and muscle tissue is an important part of your metabolism.

Carbohydrates (carbs): Carbohydrates are the quick energy of our three building blocks. They're the quick match-strike, with a brief flare of light that goes out a couple seconds later. If you take in carbs and don't use all that quick energy right away, or take in way more carbs than you'll ever use, it's eventually stored as fat. Think of lighting match after match after match, and how much trash that produces. Eating fat typically doesn't make you fat. Eating too many carbs definitely does.

How fats, proteins, and carbs fit into the Paleo diet:

Back in the day, we humans didn't have access to a lot of fat. We got our proteins primarily from animals, and the carbs we did eat came from fruit and vegetables. Fat was difficult to come by and it was a special treat because it was that slow-burning, long-lasting energy. Those delicious carbs, especially fruit with its high sugar content and starchy vegetables like potatoes, were little energy firecrackers.

That constant hunt for energy is what makes modern humans love sweet, carb-heavy foods so much. Eating quick-delivery carbs and fats literally makes our brain produce happy hormones. *Mmm,* our body says. *This winter is going to be WAY easier to survive now that I have these energy stores!*

The Paleo diet discourages those happy-producing carbs because we really don't need them. Really. We seriously do not need all that sugar. It tastes *great*, but we do not. Need. It. In case you're wondering, yes, that is the definition of an addiction. Carb addiction: it's real.

By participating in a Paleo diet, we're trimming down our meals to what we actually need, not what offers that burst of satisfaction and happy hormones that quickly fade.

For some people, getting rid of carbs and sugar is the most painful part of starting and sustaining the diet, but after a couple weeks of throttling back, you'll lose your sweet tooth and find satisfaction in healthier stuff.

Your body was designed to work in a very specific way with very specific kinds of fuel; the Paleo diet takes into account that specificity and encourages foods that fit really well within how you're actually meant to thrive.

One thing you'll notice once you're established within a Paleo diet is that it's not a "diet" at all in the traditional sense of the word. You're not limiting your intake of food; you're eliminating all the extra stuff that serves no purpose. After you get some experience and solid recipes under your belt, Paleo stops feeling like a "diet" and starts feeling like the way people should be eating.

What are the limitations of a Paleo diet?

This is the disclaimer section of our guide.

First off, if you're going to be making sweeping changes to your diet, it's recommended you discuss any plans with a medical physician or nutritionist before doing so. If you have chronic illnesses, mobility issues, a history of disordered eating, autoimmune conditions, or a restricted diet for health reasons, it's especially important you get the A-OK from a professional who's familiar with your medical history.

Second, as mentioned earlier, the Paleo diet will have the lovely side effect of slimming you down, but sharply restricting your food intake to quickly lose weight is not healthy and not recommended. Again, in order to make real, significant changes, starting slowly and learning to stick with it will be much more effective in the long run. Be patient with yourself, and don't expect your six-pack to appear in three days.

Thirdly, you'll see results much more quickly in any diet if you add an exercise program. Getting regular exercise is an important part of being a healthy person and it's absolutely recommended that you get at least half an hour of moderate exercise every day. To learn more about the importance of exercise, check out this website, created by Harvard University.

Chapter 2 Getting Started

You know what it is, you know why it works, and now you're ready to get going on your Paleo diet journey.

Surely you're very curious as to what foods are recommended for a Paleo diet. Use the charts below to double-check the ingredients in your meals and keep you on track with healthy, nourishing choices. Be sure to read the notes underneath each chart, and pay attention to the "Paleo Grey Area" chart. Once you've read through, read our tips for how to come up with a diet plan and how to conquer the grocery store.

GREEN LIGHT PALEO FOODS	
RED MEAT	Beef, deer, bison, veal, goat, rabbit, elk
OTHER MEATS & PROTEINS	Chicken, turkey, goose, quail, duck, eggs (chicken, duck, quail, goose)
FISH & SHELLFISH	Salmon, tuna, anchovies, herring, shrimp, scallops, mussels, oysters, tilapia, catfish, haddock, grouper, snapper, crab, crawfish, lobster
EVERYDAY VEGETABLES	Carrots, kale, celery, broccoli, peppers, onions, tomatoes,

	cucumbers, asparagus, Brussel sprouts, eggplant, cabbage, avocados, cauliflower, lettuce, spinach, beets, spaghetti squash, sweet potatoes, yams, turnips, mushrooms, green beans
EXOTIC VEGETABLES	Seaweed, turnip greens, beet top, bok choy, arugula, dandelion greens, artichoke, okra, watercress, fennel, rapini, radish, parsnips
FRUITS	Apples, oranges, raspberries, blueberries, blackberries, strawberries, lingberries, mango, pineapple, bananas, pomegranate, cantaloupe, honeydew melon, lemon, lime, papaya, grapes, watermelon, coconuts, dates, olives, peaches, plums, cherries, passion fruit
NUTS & SEEDS	Almonds, chia seeds, pumpkin seeds, flax seeds, walnuts, Brazil nuts, cashews, macadamia nuts, pecans, sesame seeds, hazelnuts, pine nuts
HERBS & SPICES	Mint, thyme, basil, rosemary, coriander, fennel, oregano, sage, bay, cayenne, salt, pepper, cinnamon, nutmeg, garlic, ginger, cloves, paprika, vanilla
FATS & OILS	Ghee (clarified butter), olive oil, coconut oil, avocado oil, flax seed oil, lard, rendered fat (duck, bacon), walnut oil
SWEETENERS*	Honey, Stevia, coconut sugar
NON-ANIMAL	Tofu, beans, legumes, dairy

PROTEINS** *(FOR VEGETARIANS ONLY)*	products (e.g. Kefir)
MISCELLANEOUS	Dark chocolate (at least 76% cacao)

*Though these are "whole food" sweeteners, they're still sugar and mostly-empty carbs and should be used very sparingly or not at all. Chocolate does have some nutritive properties and antioxidant benefits, but you don't need much to get those benefits. Have a small square and see how you feel.

**If you're a vegetarian and undertaking a Paleo diet, please be aware that it is ESSENTIALLY IMPOSSIBLE to consume sufficient amounts of protein from non-meat sources and also strictly adhere to a prescribed Paleo diet. If you are unable or unwilling to eat meat while on a Paleo diet, please seek out resources specifically for vegetarians. Insufficient protein and iron intake can have severe health consequences and harm your body, especially if you are very physically active. Proceed with extreme caution.

PALEO NO-GO FOODS (NOTE THAT ALCOHOL IS NOT PART OF A PALEO DIET) (SORRY)	
GRAINS & STARCHES	Bread, corn, oats, rice (white & brown), quinoa, barley, rye, buckwheat, white and russet potatoes, acorn squash, crackers, chips, pancakes, French fries, buns, toast, sandwiches, cookies, cakes, pancakes, pasta, cereal
LEGUMES	Peanuts, navy beans, black beans, chickpeas, lentils, soy products, tofu
BUTTERS	Peanut butter
OILS	Vegetable oil, canola oil, soy oils, margarine, cottonseed oil, safflower oil, peanut oil, sunflower oil, corn oil
SWEETENERS & CANDY	White sugar, corn syrup, high fructose corn syrup, refined

	sugar, brown sugar, confectioner's sugar, "Sugar in the Raw," Splenda, Truvia, artificial sweeteners (xylitol, sorbitol, saccharine, aspartame, sucralose and many others), milk chocolate, white chocolate, candy bars, gummy candies, candied fruit, licorice, mints, gum
DAIRY	Milk (skim, 2%, whole), cream, cheese (including cottage), yogurt, pudding, butter (non-clarified), ice cream, frozen yogurt, condensed milk, powdered milk, non-dairy creamer
DRINKS	Soda, diet soda, energy drinks (Red Bull, Monster etc.), apple juice, orange juice, grape juice, alcohol (beer, wine, grain alcohol), bottled coffee drinks, diet waters (Vitamin Water, Splash etc)
PROCESSED MEATS	Spam, hot dogs, deli meats, bacon with nitrates
MISCELLANEOUS	Ketchup, vinegar, store-bought vegetable chips, Clif Bars, Luna Bars, many "meal replacement" bars, protein bars and drinks, some protein powders (check for whey and added sugars), most store-bought smoothies (Jamba Juice, Smoothie King etc.)

AREA	
COFFEE & TEA	Caffeinated beverages are technically not part of a true Paleo diet. If you must drink coffee, drink it black. If you are a tea drinker, choose non-caffeinated herbal teas or green tea. No milk or sugar. One of the benefits of a Paleo diet is that your energy levels will increase; typically you will stop needing and craving caffeine after a period of time.
"NATURAL" SWEETENERS	Even "natural" sweeteners like honey and maple syrup are mostly empty calories and should be used extremely sparingly, and preferably not at all.
FRUIT & CARBOHYDRATES	Don't be nervous about carbs. Be nervous about empty, non-nutritive carbs that come from refined sugars and junk food. Fruits do have a lot of sugar in them, mostly from fructose, which is a "natural" sweetener, but they also have important vitamins that contribute to health. Watch your fruit consumption and don't overdo it.
PLANT-BASED PROTEIN SOURCES & IRON	A strict Paleo diet cuts out many of the foods that vegetarians would normally eat in order to consume healthy amounts of protein and iron. Protein-rich grains and dairy are off-limits, as are legumes and some nuts. If you

are vegetarian and starting a Paleo diet, please consider how you will incorporate enough protein in your diet to be healthful.

Putting together a plan

As they say in the military: Proper Planning and Preparation Prevents Piss-Poor Performance.

Why do we need a plan? Because a lot of why we choose to eat unhealthy food is based on convenience. We're busy/working late/have sick kids/tired and we have a lot of stuff to do. We order pizza because we're too (insert excuse) to cook real food. With the Paleo diet, you're going to **have** to find a little bit of time to make healthy choices, so that even when you're in a rush, you have something nutritious to reach for.

Planning out your meals ahead of time will ultimately save you a lot of aggravation, which is another reason why our 30-day plan in Chapter 8 is so useful—because when you're ready with your Paleo-friendly cuisine, you're not stressed about being a bad dieter. You can get on with life.

One thing that's NOT in our plan is counting calories. If you're on a Paleo diet and actually following the rules, there is absolutely no reason for you to be fixated on calories. Focus on your health and nutrition instead.

Putting together a good plan starts—you guessed it-- at the grocery store.

Conquering the Grocery Store

If you're lucky enough to have consistent access to a local farmer's market or you grow all your own produce, then hooray, going Paleo should be pretty easy for you.

But if you're like the majority of people, then you probably get your food from a plain ol' grocery store chain. It's fair to say that in many stores, more stuff isn't Paleo than is.

Why's that? Because sugar is everywhere, carbs are cheap, and we love the convenience of ready-made foods.

There's an easy trick to help keep you on the wagon and make choosing good ingredients easy: **shop the edges of the store**. If you imagine your grocery as a big box, stay away from the middle and shop the perimeter. That's typically where you'll find the fresh produce and meat, and that's where you want to be focusing your shopping energy.

A Paleo diet can actually be very economical! A couple pounds of sweet potatoes, which you can use in breakfast, lunch and dinner recipes, is a few dollars, whereas a frozen meal-in-a-bag that lasts one evening can be $7 or more.

If you want a Paleo-friendly oil that won't break the bank, coconut oil is great for everything. It has a high smoke point, mild flavor, it's full of good fats and nutrients, and it's a lot more reasonably priced than some other oils. You can also usually find it in most grocery store chains now.

If you are a regular shopper at Whole Foods or similar, it'll be a lot easier to find Paleo staples, but it'll also be more expensive. If you need something very specific, like almond flour, it can be hard to track down at WalMart or Winn Dixie or wherever you shop. For those kinds of ingredients, Whole Foods or online shopping may be your only option.

Ramping Up

Gosh, you're thinking. *There's a lot to think about and a lot to do and a LOT of stuff I can't eat...what have I gotten myself into?*

Don't panic! In our previous section, we mentioned the possibility of slowly ramping up to a prescribed Paleo diet instead of cutting out all non-Paleo foods cold turkey. You know yourself best, so you can decide which will ultimately be better for you, but if you'd like to dip your toe first, you have options.

Especially if you have a diet chock-full of the no-go foods, check out the below plans and consider starting there. Chapter 8 is written for a middle-of-the-road Paleo dieter—someone who's comfortable at least attempting to make each meal Paleo-friendly.

If you need to start slowly, that's OK! Many, many people, whether they meant to or not, have eating habits that revolve around quickly gratifying, sugar and carb-heavy foods. You're not a bad person if that's where you're coming from. But, if you're serious about changing your eating habits *permanently*, it's worth avoiding a massive shock to your body by suddenly depriving it of all its comfort foods. Slow and steady wins the race.

The most difficult things to cut out tend to be alcohol, refined sugar and quick carbs, like bread.

PLAN 1: BABY STEPS (good for regular drinkers, fast-food connoisseurs, bread and sugar lovers)

• Pay attention to when your body is asking for food because you're bored, or emotional, and when your body wants food because it's actually hungry and it's time for a meal.

• Only have one cup of coffee a day, and try to cut down on added milk and sugar.

• Limit yourself to five drinks per week (one drink = one glass of wine, one beer, or one cocktail with an ounce of hard liquor in it)

• Substitute two carb-based breakfasts a week (cereal, toast, bagel, oatmeal, toaster pastry etc.) for an egg-based meal or a fruit smoothie. (See Chapter X for breakfast recipes, including many with eggs)

• Look at the labels of what you're eating, and note when you find some kind of added sugar product. It shouldn't be hard to find—sugar is in lots of unexpected food items.

o   Cut out one super-empty food. For example, replace orange juice with seltzer water or processed sandwich meats like bologna for thinly sliced chicken breast.

•   Switch out canola or vegetable oil for olive oil, coconut oil, or ghee.

•   Instead of snacking exclusively on chips or sweet stuff, try substituting fruit leather or an ounce of Paleo-friendly nuts and a banana.

Try the above for a week, or however long you need to get comfortable and tame some of those cravings. Then, move on to the next part of the plan.

PLAN 2: THE STROLL (good for people who try and have some success at managing vices)

•   Try to only eat when you're actually hungry. Think about packing healthy snacks to tide you over between meals.

- Have one cup of coffee per day, with only a little milk, or black.

- Limit yourself to three drinks per week
- Switch out your carb-y breakfasts for a protein-filled egg-based meal, or, a fruit smoothie (try berries) with a bit of nut butter. If you must have bread with breakfast, choose a whole-grain option.

- Instead of a sandwich with slices of bread for lunch, try a wrap instead, or switch to salads with a little bit of cheese and croutons, with no bread on the side.

  o If fast food is your only option, try and get a baked potato or salad instead of a burger or sandwich.

  o Go easy on your creamy dressings.

- Stock up on healthy nuts and fruits for when the urge to snack hits you. Have some fruit leather on hand if you get desperate for sweets.

- Get rid of some more of those empty foods. Substitute yogurt with guacamole, or cookies with a small piece of dark chocolate.

- Make sure there's at least one fresh veggie on your dinner plate every night.

Hang out at the above until you feel like you can handle the changes, and then move on.

PLAN 3: POWER WALK (for people who are mostly comfortable with what a Paleo diet consists of)

- Only eat when you're hungry, and always have Paleo-friendly snacks on hand to keep you from crashing between meals.

- Try and keep your caffeine consumption to a minimum, drinking only one cup of black coffee per day, or green tea.

- Limit yourself to one drink per week.
- Keep your breakfasts protein-based, using eggs and unprocessed meats.

- If you're eating wraps for lunch, switch to salads. If you're eating salads with croutons or cheese, sub out cheese for crumbled bacon.

  - Try to sub out processed dressings (like ranch, French, Caeser) for olive oil and lemon juice.

- Sub out carb-heavy veggies (like white potatoes) for less starchy options, like yams.

If you comfortably exist as a Power Walker, then you're ready to go whole-hog. Take the final leap into eliminating the rest of those no-go foods and be fully prescribed-Paleo.

One More Thing

Yes, you're ready to eat well, be healthy, slim down and have more energy! Choosing to commit yourself to a better diet is wonderful, but you know what would make it even better?

Throwing some exercise into the mix.

If you already get at least 2.5 hours of moderate exercise every week, then terrific. Keep up the good work, and I bet once you've been Paleo for a while, you'll notice that you're performing better during your workouts.

If you are 100% sedentary, then it's time to think about adding an exercise routine. Any changes in your diet will go further, and you'll look and feel better faster, if you're coupling it with exercise. Something as simple as taking a 20-minute walk, or doing jumping jacks for a couple minutes a few times a day, will have a hugely positive impact on your overall health.

There are many free workout videos online, including introductory yoga and stretching, on YouTube and other sites like

Workout Blender. (Try Googling "Free workout routines.") You can download apps for your phone that will take you through a guided workout you can do in your living room. There are even ellipticals and recumbent bikes that fit under your desk, so you can get a little bit of exercise even while you're sitting.

You don't need a gym membership to get your heart rate up.

Make your Paleo diet as effective as it can be by exercising every day.

Chapter 3 Paleo Food Prep and Recipes

Tools

As a fresh Paleo-diet adherent, you have a new best friend, and that friend is a slow cooker.

If you're unfamiliar with them, a slow cooker, also known as a crock-pot, is an appliance that consists of a heatproof casserole dish or pot (surprise) sitting on top of an electric hot plate. Rather than boiling or frying foods to cook them, a slow cooker simmers food over long periods of time, which helps foods maintain their nutrients. If it's a good slow cooker, it'll have a timer so you can throw your ingredients in, leave it for anywhere from four to eight hours, and it'll automatically shut off, leaving you a ready-to-eat meal for when you walk in the door.

You can get a six-quart slow cooker with a timer for around $40.

Other things you'll love as a Paleoite: A food processor and a blender. Starting your day off with a smoothie or having a smoothie as a snack are fantastically healthy meal options. You can even make soups in your blender. There's nothing so quite grab-and-go as a smoothie or soup in a thermos.

If you don't have a food processor, then go get one. They're so useful for any kind of cooking, but especially in Paleo cooking. In Chapter 3, you'll notice an awful lot of our recipes use a food processor to thoroughly combine ingredients. You will never, ever regret having a food processor around.

Batch Cooking

Your other Paleo best friend is batch cooking. Using your slow cooker, you can easily make several meals' worth of something and then pack it for lunches/dinners, or freeze the leftovers.

Batch cooking means baking several chicken breasts at once, then cubing them into individual portions so you can put them in omelets, on salads, whatever. You can do this with almost any kind of Paleo food—do a big pan of roast vegetables and keep some to add to other meals; eat the rest for dinner. Having everything ready to assemble into a meal is a great way to keep you honest. And, in a pinch, if it's the only thing in your fridge, you can always just eat some cubed chicken to tide you over while you make something else.

One of the best things to have in your freezer is bags of vegetables and vegetable medleys. Go for the ones that are only vegetables, no added sauces or, salts or grains. If you're desperate, in between shopping trips, or just don't feel like roasting veggies, get out one of your microwavable frozen veggie bags and voila. Serve it with a few ounces of meat and you've got the Paleo equivalent of fast food.

Paleo Substitution Hacks

As you get comfortable with Paleo recipes and cooking, you'll notice Paleo items appearing in place of other items that are less healthy. Sometimes, you'll find a recipe you really love, but it has some no-go items in it. There are often substitutions you can make to keep the integrity of the recipe without being unfaithful to your diet.

The recipe calls for...	Use this instead...
White flour	Coconut flour, tapioca flour, almond flour*
Spaghetti	Spaghetti squash
Rice	Cauliflower (finely chopped)**
Potato chips	Thinly-sliced sweet potatoes or kale
Soy sauce	Coconut aminos***
Milk	Coconut milk, almond milk****
Sugar	Honey
Bread	Iceberg lettuce

*Different flours cause foods to cook/bake/rise differently, so be ready to experiment with amounts and types.

**Cauliflower is a great stand-in for many carbs. You can also use it to make pizza dough by putting it in a food processor and adding some almond flour.

***Aminos are a soy-free, wheat-free liquid that have the same salty taste as regulation non-Paleo soy sauce.

****If you're baking, use coconut milk instead of animal milk. If you're cooking, try almond milk instead of animal milk.

Chapter 4: Paleo Snacks

First off, there's no hard and fast rule that says YOU MUST EAT THREE MEALS A DAY AND THEY SHALL BE BREAKFAST, LUNCH AND DINNER. In fact, that's kind of stupid. A lot of people function much better if they're able to eat five or six small meals a day rather than three big ones. Keeping a bit of fuel in your tank maintains your metabolism and pays out energy more efficiently.

If you're a three-meals-a-day person, then you're probably also a guilty snacker.

Going back to the idea of choosing foods out of convenience, consider the snack:

The need for snacks and dieter's inability to satisfy that urge with Paleo food is one reason why people get fed up and quit.

Let's consider: it's 7 PM. You're stuck at the office. Or, you're stuck in traffic. Or, you can't get the kids organized. Or, you're bored or had a bad day. Lo and behold, you remember that in your desk/glove box/bag/freezer, you have a bag of chips/candy bar/something in a wrapper. So you eat it.

That last one in particular—being bored or emotional—is a killer. We humans tend to eat junk when we're emotional because of that rush of happy hormones from sugar makes us feel a little bit better, at least temporarily.

When you're on a Paleo diet and you have an undeniable urge to shove something in your mouth and mindlessly eat, what are your options?

First of all, **stop and think why you want to eat**. Is it because you're actually hungry? If so, then proceed to the next step. If not, then drink a bunch of water and try to do something else. If you're not hungry, you don't need to eat. Once you do that enough times, your body will stop crying wolf and you'll lose the random cravings.

When doing your batch cooking, make a bunch of these little tidbits and have them in single-serving portions so you're ready when you need sustenance between meals. Remember, more frequent, smaller meals are a good thing.

PALEO SNACKS		
A piece of fruit, like a banana	Kale or sweet potato chips	Hard boiled egg
An ounce of nuts (not peanuts!)	One piece of dark chocolate	Jerky
Smoothie	A couple bites of leftovers	Tuna with guacamole
Roasted pumpkin seeds	Paleo energy bars (recipe below)	Almond butter and celery
Chocolate-covered bacon (yes!)	Coconut-crusted chicken	Cauliflower "crackers"

I've found that bananas are basically the perfect snack food. They come in their own wrapper, they're filled with potassium and other excellent vitamins, they're inexpensive, and they're a single serving. There's less snack guesswork eating a banana than there is in a "handful" of nuts. Eggs are also a great choice because they have a lot of protein, which quiets hungry bellies quickly, and helps you feel full for longer.

A lot of people enjoy having a grab-and-go option that isn't just a banana. Here's an easy recipe for Paleo energy bars:

No-Bake Paleo-Friendly Energy Bars	Makes 12-15 bars
Ingredients	**Directions**
<ul><li>1/3 cup dark chocolate cocoa powder</li><li>1 cup dates with pits removed</li><li>¼ finely-chopped flax seed</li><li>½ cup unsalted nuts of your choice (almonds, macadamia, etc.)</li><li>½ cup second unsalted nut of your choice (Brazil nut, walnut etc.)</li><li>½ cup dried berries like cranberry, (no added sugar, no raisins)</li><li>1 tsp. vanilla</li><li>1 tsp. cinnamon</li><li>1.5 tbsp. coconut oil</li></ul>	1. Add pitted dates to a food processor and blend until they make a gooey, sticky paste. If they're not getting gooey, add a little bit of warm water. 2. Add finely chopped or ground flax seeds, cocoa powder, vanilla and cinnamon, and coconut oil. Use the "pulse" setting to blend them together, but don't liquefy them. 3. Add your half cups of nuts and pulse a few more times until chopped. 4. Stir in your dried berries. Do not use the food processor! 5. Have a baking sheet with parchment paper ready. Scoop out your mixture and, using a big spoon lightly oiled with coconut oil, mash down the mix until it's about a half inch thick and evenly spread. 6. Cover them with plastic wrap and put them in the fridge to set for at least an hour. 7. Remove the plastic wrap and cut them into squares, 3x4 or 3x5. 8. Eat!

Dates are a great Paleo-friendly food that can be used in snacks and desserts. You can wrap them with bacon for a delicious appetizer, or process them to make a sweet, sticky, almost toffee-like substances that works as a good sugar sub in many recipes.

Chapter 5: Basic Meals Anyone Can Master

You're just starting out and you need some practice mastering this Paleo cooking thing. Start here with these foolproof (though basic) recipes that are quick, easy, satisfying, and don't require a lot of fancy stuff. You'll notice they feature a lot of eggs—that's because eggs are such a great source of protein, and incredibly versatile.

If you're a lazy cook (like me), you might never progress much further than these recipes, which is totally fine. If you are happy with simple meals, then care of this list, your life just got a lot easier.

Blank Canvas Omelet	10 minutes, 1 serving
Ingredients	**Directions**
<ul><li>3 eggs (whites and yolks)</li><li>½ tbsp. ghee or coconut oil</li><li>Salt and pepper to taste<ul><li>OPTIONAL</li></ul></li></ul>	*Note: the sky is the limit with this omelet. If you're feeling lazy, just do the eggs. If you have some leftover meat or veggies, throw it in.*

• ¼ cup almond milk or coconut milk • MEATS (must be cooked): diced chicken, ham, bacon, sausage, prosciutto, canned tuna • VEGGIES (cooked or uncooked depending on preference): spinach, kale, mushrooms, avocado, onion, tomato, sweet potato, peppers, garlic	1. Combine eggs, salt and pepper in a bowl and beat well (if you prefer a fluffier omelet, separate whites and eggs, beat whites until stiff, then combine with yolk) 2. Heat a small pan with angled sides (easier to made the omelet slide out) and let your ghee or oil heat, but not overheat 3. Pour in your egg mixture and tilt pan so it's evenly spread (if you want a denser omelet, use a smaller pan) 4. If you're adding optional ingredients, do so while the eggs are still slightly runny 5. Cook to desired doneness, and then serve.

I like a construction metaphor when it comes to eggs and omelets in a Paleo diet: eggs are your steel beams and wood, and you can combine them in many different ways to build different things. Then, (to extend the metaphor) do all the finish work using the fun stuff—in this case, vegetables and spices. Omelets don't have to be savory, either. If you make a very thin omelet, almost like a crepe, you can add berries and even a bit of melted dark chocolate. Your imagination is your only limit when it comes to omelets.

Oven Baked Eggs	15 minutes prep, 5 minutes bake, 4 servings
Ingredients	**Directions**
<ul><li>8 eggs</li><li>OPTIONAL: ¼ cup coconut milk</li><li>2 tbsp. ghee</li><li>¼ - ½ cup chopped bacon</li><li>¼ - ½ cup mushrooms</li><li>¼ - ½ cup diced tomatoes</li><li>¼ cup diced onion</li><li>1 cup sliced zucchini rounds</li><li>Salt & pepper to taste</li></ul>	1. In a large fry pan, add ghee and cook onions until translucent, then add pieces of bacon; cook for 2-3 minutes; add mushroom and tomatoes, cook until just soft, then remove from heat and set aside. 2. Use your oven's "broil" setting 3. In a large bowl, beat together your eggs and add salt and pepper to taste 4. Take a pie dish or casserole dish (eyeball size—you don't want egg mixture spread too thin or to be overflowing) and add eggs 5. Take your cooked veggies and meats and stir throughout the eggs. Use ¼ cup if you want the eggs to shine through, or add full amount for a very dense, hearty dish 6. Top with rounds of zucchini 7. Bake for 3-4 minutes, watching carefully for

	browning around the edges. If you have more ingredients, cook 4-5 minutes. 8. Serve!

Like our omelet, oven-baked eggs, or frittata, is another great vehicle for any and everything Paleo. You can substitute any kind of veggie in frittatas, or different kinds of meat like chicken, beef, or even seafood.

Crockpot Pulled Pork	Time: 8 hours
Ingredients	**Directions**
• 4 lbs. pork loin or shoulder • ½ cup apple cider vinegar • ¼ cup raw honey • 1 tbsp. coconut oil • 2 cloves garlic • 1 tbsp. coconut aminos • 1 tbsp. thyme • ½ tbsp. onion & garlic powder • Salt & pepper • OPTIONAL: mustard (check labels for additives)	1. Mix together honey, thyme, onion and garlic powders and mustard, if you're using it 2. Add coconut aminos and apple cider vinegar to spices and combine well 3. Lightly salt and pepper the loin 4. Coat the bottom of the pot with the coconut oil 5. Place the meat in the slow cooker and rub the spice/cider mixture on top 6. Peel garlic cloves and put them whole in with the meat 7. Set your slow cooker for 8 hours on the low setting 8. Once done, pull apart the meat using your fingers or two forks to shred it 9. Serve! NOTE: you can make this recipe

	using beef instead of pork—add 2 cups of beef stock, and substitute balsamic vinegar for apple cider vinegar

Hopefully crock-pot pulled pork will help you to see just how fantastic slow cookers can be. You can use many different kinds of meat, as noted in the bottom of the recipe—try using beef instead of pork. You can also use less meat and leave room for hard root vegetables, like sweet potatoes, onions, carrots, turnips and parsnips, which will cook delightfully and make this an even better one pot meal.

Grilled Veggies	**10 minutes prep, 30 minutes bake, 1-8 servings**
Ingredients	**Directions**
NOTE: you can scale this recipe up or down depending on how much you'd like to cook at once and how big your roasting pans are • 4 large carrots • 4 turnips • 1 yellow onion • 1 lb. Brussel sprouts • 1 large sweet potato • 1 head of broccoli • 1 head of cauliflower	1. Preheat your oven to 400 degrees 2. Chop your veggies into rough chunks, about 1x1"—don't make them too small, as they'll cook too quickly and turn to mush 3. Place your veggies in a large bowl with the 2 tbsp. of coconut oil and add salt and pepper. Toss until they're evenly coated with oil and condiments 4. Take a large roasting pan and rub the bottom with coconut oil 5. Place veggies on your pan in

• 2 tbsp. coconut oil • Salt & pepper	one even layer 6. Bake for 30 minutes, or until broccoli is browned and the sweet potatoes can be easily penetrated with a fork

I think grilled veggies are one of the best meals for a Paleo diet. First of all, all of those veggies are cheap, you can get them almost anywhere, and you can make loads and loads of them at once, so you always have a little container of roast veggies waiting for you. Try any kinds of vegetables; though be warned that those with higher water content, like tomatoes, can get very, very soft and messy. You can also dress up this recipe a bit more with things like fresh rosemary, fennel or thyme.

Chili	10 minutes prep, 40 minutes cook, 4 servings
Ingredients	**Directions**
• 4 cups of roast shredded turkey meat (or leftover chicken or pork) • 4 large carrots • 1 bell pepper • 1 yellow onion • 2 large tomatoes	1. Dice your vegetables and shred your meat, if it isn't already in small pieces. Finely chop the garlic. 2. In a large pot heated on medium-high, add your ghee or lard, garlic, onions and carrots, and cook 2 minutes until beginning to soften

• 4 cloves garlic • 1 tbsp. tomato paste or 2 tbsp. tomato sauce (make sure sauce has no sugar) • 1 cup chicken stock (not broth—check ingredients) • OPTIONAL: chili powder to taste • 1 tbsp. cumin • 1 tsp. oregano • Salt & pepper • 1 tbsp. ghee or lard	3. Add bell peppers and cook for 1 more minute 4. Add all spices and stir until aromatic 5. Add tomato paste or sauce, tomatoes, stock, all spices, and shredded meat 6. Briefly bring to a boil, and then leave the pot uncovered on a low setting for about 30 minutes or to taste, then serve

You can't go wrong with chili. It freezes well and it requires basically no work besides some chopping and stirring. Plus, you really don't need to invest in any kind of special ingredients to make it delicious. This recipe is great to use with leftover meat. If you have a roast chicken or turkey you have mostly picked over, pull off the rest of that meat and throw it in a chili.

Crock-pot Apples and Cabbage	10 minutes prep, 6-8 hours cook, 6 servings
Ingredients	Directions

Ingredients	Instructions
• 2-3 large Granny Smith apples (depending on size of your slow cooker) • 1 head of cabbage • 1 yellow onion • ½ cup apple cider vinegar • 2 tbsp. mustard • Salt & pepper • 1 tbsp. ghee or coconut oil	1. Coat your crockpot with your oil or ghee 2. Rough chop your apples and cabbage and add to pot 3. Quarter your onion and add to pot 4. In a small bowl, combine apple cider vinegar, mustard, salt and pepper and mix well 5. Pour the mixture over the cabbage, apples and onion, and mix well 6. Cook on low setting for 6 hours; if you can, stir every couple of hours. If, after 6 hours cabbage is not tender, cook for another 2 hours on low 7. Serve with your leftover pulled pork

I love this recipe because it's a bit sweet, with nice textures, and again, pure crock pot genius. This goes so well with pulled pork. If you have a large crock-pot (6 quarts or more), it's easy to make a lot of this and stretch it out for many meals.

Chapter 6: Heartier Fare

You've mastered the basics, and you're ready to branch out. Try adding these delicious recipes into your Paleo repertoire!

BREAKFAST: Do NOT skip breakfast! Many of these recipes are grab-and-go, or you can do double portions for breakfast and another for lunch.

All-day Energy Breakfast Skillet	10 minutes prep, 10 minutes cook, 2 servings
Ingredients	**Directions**
<ul><li>1 sweet large potato</li><li>1 cup bell pepper</li><li>1 cup chopped onion</li><li>Handful of spinach</li><li>1 large tomato</li><li>1.5 tsps. olive oil or coconut oil</li><li>2 garlic cloves</li><li>2 pre-cooked chicken sausage links</li><li>4 pieces bacon (cooked)</li><li>Salt & pepper</li></ul>	1. Rough chop sweet potato, pepper, and tomato. Make sure potato is chopped small enough that it will cook through easily 2. Dice onion and finely chop or crush garlic 3. Slice pre-cooked chicken links into rounds and rough chop bacon 4. Heat olive or coconut oil in a large skillet or fry pan 5. Add onion, garlic, and sweet potato; let cook, stirring occasionally, until sweet potato begins to

	soften. Season with salt and pepper to taste. 6. Add bell peppers, stir briefly, then add tomato 7. Add meats and simmer, covered, for 3 minutes 8. Add spinach and stir until wilted, then immediately remove from heat 9. Serve!

*Adapted from *Fast Paleo's* Loaded Paleo Breakfast Hash recipe

Biscuits for the Flour-Challenged	5 minutes prep, 20 minutes bake, 8 servings
Ingredients	**Directions**
• 3 cups almond flour • 2 eggs • 2 tbsp. honey • ¼ tsp. salt • 1 tsp. baking soda • 1 tbsp. lemon juice	1. Preheat the oven to 325 degrees 2. Combine the almond flour, salt and baking soda in a bowl, gently combining 3. Make a well in the middle and add the eggs, lemon juice and honey 4. Stir with a large spoon to combine the mixture into a heavy dough 5. Divide the dough into 8 equal-sized pieces and flatten each one to 1½ inches. Use the back of a metal spoon as your flattener 6. Arrange the biscuits on a parchment paper-lined cookie sheet and bake for 20 minutes or until cooked through and lightly browned

*Adapted from *CavemanDietBlog.com*

Grab-and-Go Eggy Muffins	10 minutes prep, 15 minutes cook, 12 servings
Ingredients	**Directions**
<ul><li>6 eggs</li><li>½ large tomato</li><li>4 small mushroom caps</li><li>4 strips of cooked bacon</li><li>1 tsp. roasted chopped garlic or garlic salt</li><li>2 tbsp. ghee or aerosolized coconut oil</li></ul>	1. Preheat oven to 350 degrees and get out a 12-cup muffin tin 2. Dice mushrooms and briefly sauté in a small fry pan over medium heat. Remove once they're soft 3. Crack eggs into a large bowl and beat them together 4. Chop up your tomatoes and bacon 5. Add all ingredients in with the eggs 6. Grease your tin to prevent sticking and add contents of the bowl into the cups. Fill about 2/3rd full 7. Bake for 15 minutes then remove with a silicone spatula

*Adapted from *Not too Shabby Gabby*

Wholly Avocados	5 minutes prep, 20 minutes cook, 2 servings
Ingredients	**Directions**
<ul><li>1 avocado</li><li>2 eggs</li><li>Salt & pepper</li></ul>	1. Preheat oven to 400 degrees 2. Cut avocado in half and remove the pit 3. Crack an egg into the middle of each avocado half 4. Sprinkle with salt and pepper 5. Bake for 20 minutes or until egg is your desired consistency 6. Eat with a spoon

*Adapted from *Swirls of Flavor* blog

Quick Blueberry Breakfast Smoothie	5 minutes, 1 serving
Ingredients	**Directions**
<ul><li>1 cup frozen blueberries</li><li>1 green apple</li><li>1 frozen banana</li><li>¾ cup fresh-squeezed cup orange juice (no added sugar)</li><li>¼ cup almond milk (no added sugar)</li></ul>	1. Put all your ingredients in a blender and blend until smooth 2. If desired, add ice to thin, or add flax seed powder to thicken

*Adapted from *VeggieSouls.com*

No-bake Nut Bars	10 minutes prep, 2 hours set, 4 servings
Ingredients	**Directions**
<ul><li>1 cup almonds</li><li>1 cup cashew nuts</li><li>½ cup shredded coconut (no added sugar)</li><li>¼ cup honey</li><li>¼ tsp. salt</li></ul>	1. Get out your food processor and finely chop the almonds and cashews 2. Add the coconut flakes and pulse one or two more times until just combined. Switch mixture to a bowl and add honey and salt 3. Line a baking sheet with parchment paper and press out your mixture until it's flat and about a half inch thick 4. Chill in the fridge until it's set, about 2 hours. 5. Cut into squares

*Adapted from *PaleoPlan.com*

Paleo Pancakes	5 minutes prep, 10 minutes cook, 1 serving
Ingredients	**Directions**
Note: this recipe is for one serving. Triple or quadruple the recipe as you like. • 1 egg • 1 ripe banana • 2 ½ tsps. coconut flour • 1 pinch baking powder • 1 pinch cinnamon • ½ tbsp. ghee	1. Mash the banana very well 2. Add all the ingredients (except the coconut oil) in a bowl and mix 3. Add the ghee to a fry pan and ladle about a quarter cup of the mixture into the pan (use more batter if you want larger pancakes) 4. Cook until golden brown, then flip and repeat 5. Serve with ghee and maple syrup

*Adapted from *PaleoGrubs.com*

LUNCH AND DINNER OPTIONS:

The below can be used for lunches or dinners. Many of these freeze well and will last for a long time if you cook them in batches. Bon appetite!

Zucchini Chips	15 minutes prep, 1.5-2 hours bake, 5 servings
Ingredients	**Directions**
<ul><li>1 medium zucchini (or more)</li><li>1 tbsp. olive or coconut oil</li><li>¼ tsp. onion powder</li><li>¼ tsp. garlic powder</li><li>¼ tsp. salt</li></ul>	1. Preheat your oven to 250 degrees 2. A mandolin is recommended to get the zucchinis sliced to an even thinness—about ¼ inch thick 3. Each zucchini will produce between 80-100 chips. Plan accordingly 4. Press zucchini slices between paper towels to make sure any excess water is removed 5. Line baking sheets (you may need more than 1 depending on the size of your sheet) with parchment paper and lightly spray with aerosolized oil 6. Lay out slices of zucchini and sprinkle with seasonings and salt 7. Lightly mist with oil 8. Bake until crispy, but not overly browned, between 1-2 hours. Flip half way through

*Adapted from Skinny Mom

Note: these chips do not store well (they get soggy very quickly) so it's not recommended that you make more than you can eat in a couple days.

Paleo-friendly Coconut Shrimp	5 minutes prep, 12 minutes cook, 4

	servings
Ingredients	**Directions**
• 1 ½ lbs. large fresh shrimp (wild) • 2 eggs • 2 cups shredded coconut • ¼ tsp. black pepper • ½ tsp. salt • coconut oil	1. Peel and devein your shrimp, leaving the tail so you can easily pick up the shrimp 2. Crack two eggs into a bowl (this will be for dredging your shrimp) and beat well, then add salt and pepper 3. Layer shredded unsweetened coconut on a plate 4. Dip your shrimp in the eggs, coating thoroughly, then roll them in the coconut. Set them aside 5. Heat your coconut oil for frying; pour oil into a pan until you have a depth that will be enough to float the shrimp while they cook 6. Cook a few shrimp at a time and, using long tongs, flip them after 3 or so minutes 7. Place cooked shrimp on a paper towel and let them drain/cool.

*Adapted from *PaleoGrubs.com*

No Wrap Turkey Wrap	10 minutes for prep, 10 minutes to cook, 8 servings
Ingredients	**Directions**

Ingredients	Directions
- 1 lb. ground turkey - 8 whole Boston/iceberg lettuce leaves - 1 cup carrots - 2 cloves garlic - 1 tbsp. fresh ginger - 3 tbsp. lime juice - 3 tbsp. ghee - ¼ tsp. salt	1. Shred carrots and ginger, and mince garlic 2. Heat ghee in a large fry pan 3. Add carrots, ginger, and garlic, and salt, and cook until fragrant 4. Add ground turkey to pan and cook thoroughly 5. Spoon out cooked turkey mixture evenly into 8 lettuce leaves 6. Sprinkle top with lime juice 7. Eat!

Breadless BLT	20 minutes of prep, 15 minutes of cooking, 4 servings
Ingredients	**Directions**
- 8 slices cooked bacon - 4 chicken breasts - ¼ cup Paleo mayonnaise (recipe below) - 2 tomatoes - 1 cup baby spinach - 2 tbsps. fresh basil	1. Wrap your 4 raw chicken breast between two pieces of plastic wrap and using a meat tenderizer, thin them to an even ½ inch 2. Rub the chicken with coconut oil, salt and pepper, and grill for 4-5 minutes or until internal temperature is at least 172 degrees 3. Slice the tomatoes into rounds 4. "Butterfly" or cut chicken breasts long-wise until they resemble two pieces of bread with an edge connected 5. Spread the inside of the chicken with Paleo mayo, layer on bacon, tomato and basil 6. Eat like a sandwich, minus the bread

*Adapted from *ScrappyGeek.com*

Note: the above recipe with a "bread" of chicken breast works well for any kind of sandwich you might want to prepare

Paleo Mayonnaise	20 minutes
Ingredients	**Directions**
<ul><li>2 egg yolks</li><li>½ cup olive oil</li><li>½ cup coconut oil</li><li>3 tsp. lemon juice</li><li>Salt & pepper</li><li>OPTIONAL: 1 tsp. mustard</li></ul>	1. In a blender (preferable) or food processor, combine the egg yolks and a third of the lemon juice (and mustard if you're using it) 2. While still blending on low, add a bit of oil to the mixture very slowly (a tsp. at a time), making sure that what you've added has already been thoroughly combined before adding any more 3. As you continue to add oil and blend, eventually the mixture will begin to thicken and you can begin to add the rest of the oils more quickly 4. Once it's thick, add your remaining lemon juice and salt and pepper to taste 5. Store it in a mason or other re-sealable jar in the refrigerator

*Adapted from *PaleoLeap.com*

Cauliflower "Tortillas"	15 minutes prep, 15 minutes cook, 6 servings
Ingredients	**Directions**

Ingredients	Instructions
• 1 head cauliflower • 2 eggs • ½ tsp. oregano • Salt & pepper • OPTIONAL: spices for flavoring, like paprika, chili powder, rosemary etc.	1. Preheat your oven to 375 degrees 2. Boil a pot of water (used for steaming; don't need much water) 3. Blend or food process your cauliflower until it resembles coarse "flour" 4. Put your blended cauliflower into a fine-mesh strainer and suspend it over the boiling water so it steams, for about 5 minutes 5. Let the cauliflower cool, and then using cheesecloth or a dish cloth (paper towel is NOT recommended), wrap the cooked cauliflower into a small satchel and squeeze as much of the water out as you can. Repeat as many times as necessary to get your "flour" as dry as possible 6. Put the cauliflower in a bowl and add the eggs and spices, stirring until it's complete combined 7. On a parchment-lined baking sheet, divide the cauliflower mixture into six equal parts and flatten them into tortilla-sized circles (about 5" diameter) 8. Bake them for 8 minutes, then flip, then bake for 4 more 9. If you're not going to use right away, reheat in a pan on low heat. These freeze well.

*Adapted from *PaleoLeap.com*

Note: These "tortillas" can be used in the place of anything that requires a wrap or bread.

Basic Brussel Sprouts	10 minutes prep, 40 minutes cook, 4 servings
Ingredients	**Directions**
<ul><li>2 lbs. Brussel sprouts</li><li>2 garlic cloves</li><li>1 tbsp. olive oil</li><li>1 tsp. balsamic vinegar</li><li>Salt & pepper</li></ul>	1. Preheat oven to 400 degrees 2. Slice Brussel sprouts into halves, and discard the woody stems 3. Finely mince the garlic cloves 4. Add sprouts and garlic into a bowl, and pour on balsamic and olive oil. Stir to coat 5. Add sprouts to a baking dish and cook uncovered for 40 minutes or until the sprouts are starting to brown

Easiest Crockpot Whole Chicken	5 minutes of prep, 4 hours of cooking, 6-8 servings
Ingredients	**Directions**
<ul><li>1 whole chicken (weight depends on size of slow cooker; approx. 5 lb. bird)</li><li>½ tbsp. paprika</li><li>½ tsp. salt</li><li>½ tsp. black pepper</li><li>¼ tsp. garlic powder</li><li>¼ tsp. onion powder</li></ul>	6. Dress your chicken, getting rid of gizzards, loose skin and fat. Tie legs with butcher's twine if you need to 7. Grease your crockpot with coconut oil 8. Rub your chicken with the spices 9. Set your crock pot to high and let sit for 4 hours

• 2 tbsp. coconut oil	10. Check to make sure internal temperature of chicken has reached at least 165 degrees before stopping the cooking process 11. Carve and enjoy!
Orange Chicken	**15 minutes prep, 15 minutes cook, 4 servings**
Ingredients	**Directions**
• 1 lb. chicken breast • 2 tbsp. coconut oil • Juice from 2 oranges • 1 tbsp. orange zest • 1 tsp. fresh ginger • 3 tbsp. coconut aminos • 1 tsp. garlic chili sauce	1. Cut your chicken breasts into bite-sized pieces and mince ginger 2. In a large fry pan, heat coconut oil on medium-high heat and add the chicken breast, cooking until golden brown (5 minutes) 3. Put together orange juice and zest, ginger, coconut aminos and chili sauce, and blend well 4. After chicken has finished browning, add the orange mixture into the chicken and cook until high until the liquid ingredients are beginning to boil off 5. Stir to keep the mixture from burning; once the sauce has thickened to your desired consistency, remove and serve

*Adapted from *FakeGinger.com*

Chicken & Chipotle Stuffed Sweet Potatoes	**20 minutes prep, 40 minutes cooking, 8**

	servings
Ingredients	**Directions**
• 4 large sweet potatoes • 1 lb. chicken breast or tenders • 1-2 chipotle peppers (or more if you like spice) • 1 bag of spinach • 3 tbsp. coconut oil • Salt & pepper	1. Poke your sweet potatoes with a fork and either bake them in a 450 degree oven until they're soft (around 40 minutes) or microwave them on high until soft (about 5 minutes each) 2. Dice the chipotle peppers; if you dislike spice, omit the peppers entirely 3. While sweet potatoes cook, dice your chicken breast, add the peppers, and cook on medium high in a fry pan, until just done. Set chicken aside 4. In the same fry pan, wilt the spinach, leaving it bright green 5. Cut your sweet potatoes in half and scoop out the middle, leaving 8 shells behind 6. Assemble your potato shells with the chicken and peppers; layer spinach on top and drizzle with leftover coconut oil 7. Place in oven for 5-10 minutes, then serve

Crockpot Beef and Broccoli	**15 minutes prep, 5+ hours cook, 4 servings**
Ingredients	**Directions**

• 1 lb. boneless chuck roast • 3 cups broccoli florets • 1 apple • ½ cup beef stock • 1/3 cup coconut aminos • 1/3 cup raw honey • 3 garlic cloves	12. Slice your roast into thin pieces, mince the garlic and rough chop the apples 13. Add beef stock, coconut aminos, honey, apples and garlic to the slow cooker and stir together 14. Add the thin-sliced pieces of roast and set the timer for 4-5 hours on low 15. 30 minutes before the beef is finished cooking, add the fresh broccoli florets 16. Serve!

*Adapted from *PaleoLeap.com*

DESSERTS: You didn't think there was such a thing as a Paleo dessert, did you? Thank *goodness* you're wrong. Some are even no-bake recipes, like Paleo chocolate mousse.

If you're doing baking, as mentioned earlier, Paleo-safe flours tend to behave a little bit differently than traditional gluten/wheat flours. Some, like almond flour, have a bit of a flavor (which is delicious) and are a little more grainy and heavy; some, like tapioca flour, are very fluffy and almost sweet, but you need a lot of it to hold up your recipe.

In general, don't expect Paleo baked goods to rise like traditional ones, but they'll still be delicious and hey, dessert is dessert, right?

Chocolate (Avocado) Mousse	5 minutes prep, 30 minutes chill, 2 servings
Ingredients	**Directions**
<ul><li>2 ripe avocados</li><li>2 bananas</li><li>½ cup unsweetened cocoa powder</li><li>2 tsp. vanilla extract</li><li>½ tsp. cinnamon</li><li>1/3 cup coconut milk</li></ul>	1. Half the avocado, de-pit, and cube 2. Put all ingredients into a food processor and blend until creamy 3. Chill in the fridge for half an hour 4. Serve!

*Adapted from *ToSimplyInspire.com*

Paleo Cinnamon Cookies	15 minutes prep, 10 minutes cook, makes

	20 cookies
Ingredients	**Directions**
• 2 cups almond flour • 1/8 tsp. sea salt • 1/8 tsp. baking soda • 1 tsp. ground cinnamon • ¼ cup palm shortening • 2 tbsps. honey • ½ cup coconut sugar	1. Preheat your oven to 350 degrees 2. Put flour, baking soda, cinnamon and salt into a food processor and pulse until just combined 3. Slowly add in honey and shortening 4. Take a table spoon and scoop out a serving of the dough; roll it in the coconut sugar and put it on a parchment-lined baking sheet 5. Flatten the balls of dough until they're about ¼ inch thick 6. Cook for 5-7 minutes or until golden brown 7. OPTIONAL: sprinkle a little more cinnamon over the top of the cookies once they're done

*Adapted from ElanasPantry.com

Paleo Dark Chocolate Brownies	**15 minutes prep, 20 minutes bake, 8 brownies**
Ingredients	**Directions**
• 1 cup almond flour • 4 ounces 100% cacao baking chocolate (no sugar, no	1. Preheat your oven to 350 degrees 2. Put dry ingredients in a food processor and mix until combined 3. Add chocolate and dates; chop until very fine

milk)	4. Add eggs and pulse until well combined
• 3 eggs	
• ½ tsp. vanilla extract	5. Add in vanilla extract, stevia and coconut oil
• ½ tsp. Stevia	
• ½ cup fresh pitted dates	6. Grease an 8x8 baking tin and spoon in brownie mixture
• ¼ tsp. salt	
• ¼ tsp. baking soda	7. Bake for 20 minutes
	8. Let cool for a VERY LONG TIME—up to a couple hours—before cutting
• ½ cup coconut oil	
	9. Serve!

*Adapted from ElanasPantry.com

Chapter 7: Your 14-day Jump Start

Congrats on making it this far! You've (hopefully) learned a lot and you know what you're getting yourself into. Ideally, you're not too terrified about what the Paleo "diet" entails anymore, because you've seen that it's less a diet and more a way of just getting rid of stuff our bodies don't need.

For the next two weeks, focus on incorporating the recipes from this book into your breakfasts, lunches and dinners. Keep noticing why you're choosing to eat. (Am I hungry, or am I bored or emotional?) If you slip up, it's OK; don't beat yourself up. Forgive yourself, and move on. Significant change can be hard, but it's worth it.

For your first week of Paleo, use the recipes provided in this guide to get you started. In subsequent weeks, keep recipes you enjoy in rotation and experiment with the suggested meals and ingredients for other spots.

WEEK ONE	Breakfast	Lunch	Dinner	Snacks
Sunday	Paleo pancakes	Cauliflower tortillas with crockpot beef	Chicken and chipotle stuffed sweet potatoes	Jerky and a piece of fruit
Monday	Avocado with egg in the middle	Roast vegetables and crockpot beef	Crockpot chicken with roast vegetables	1 oz. Brazil nuts, 1 banana
Tuesday	Breakfast skillet	Leftover chicken in lettuce wraps	Coconut shrimp and garlic broccoli	Blueberry smoothie in 2 servings
Wednesday	Avocado with egg in the middle	Leftover coconut shrimp and garlic broccoli	Chili with leftover chicken	No-bake nut bars
Thursday	Leftover breakfast skillet	No-bread BLT	Crockpot pulled pork, cabbage and apples	Zucchini chips, no-bake nut bar

Friday	Breakfast smoothie	Cabbage and apples with baked chicken	Leftover chili	Fruit salad in 2 servings
Saturday	Scrambled eggs and bacon	Pulled pork in lettuce wraps	Crockpot beef and broccoli	Blueberry smoothie in 2 servings

Now go enjoy your slimmer, healthier, more energetic life!

www.ingramcontent.com/pod-product-compliance
Lightning Source LLC
Chambersburg PA
CBHW071236280526
45787CB00002B/946